A Look Back

Book 4

David E. Wade, M.D.

DEDICATION

To Peggy, to my parents, and to my sisters.

Contents of Book 1:   Page

Contents of Book 2:   Page

Contents of Book 3:   Page

Contents of Book 4:   Page

ACKNOWLEDGMENTS

To the University of Cincinnati College of Medicine where I received a superb medical education, and to my wife, Peggy, who helped in innumerable ways.

i

Preface.

This book is an attempt to change the way doctors establish a diagnosis. It became obvious during my internship that most doctors try to recall from memory the various possible causes for a patient's illness. However, the memory is fallible. Consequently, many patients are misdiagnosed and the results can be disastrous.

Most of my professional career has been trying to correct the problem. This book describes my efforts, the frustrations, the disbeliefs, and the obstacles of that endeavor.

Some of the vignettes are medically instructive; some are merely fun to recall. I hope the reader enjoys the book and learns something from it.

"Satus est initius mederi quam fini." (It is better to doctor at the beginning than at the end.)   Erasmus

Chapter 15 My Medical Practice.

I opened a solo practice of medicine at the largest private hospital in the country. Those early years were somewhat difficult, but not necessarily unusual for a doctor just starting a medical practice. Doing it alone as a solo practitioner was I guess the most difficult. Peggy and I did not have a support group, a back up of other doctors and their wives with whom to discuss the ups and downs of a medical practice.

Peggy worked at the office the first three years, and this of course made her aware of the usual stress of a medical practice. Most patients were wonderful. Some were terrible. However even one terrible patient in 20 wonderful patients can ruin your day.

Peggy was the secretary, the office manager, the bookkeeper, the CFO, the insurance preparer, the fee collector, and had to be there from nine to five. One day after work our car wouldn't start. Peggy cried a little. Tough day. Car broken down. Trying to get a solo practice started. Lonely.

I remember looking at the inside of an office closet. Taped to the door were lists of equipment, stationary, and supplies. Peggy prepared the lists as a reminder of what, and when to reorder things. Neat lists. Long lists. Her dedication to the job. Her devotion. Her determination to do it and to do it right. We obviously made it, but those first years were a little frustrating.

Finally, after having gone through three or four secretaries, we hired Mrs. Winston who had been the secretary for Peggy's father. Mrs. Winston did everything except the books. Peggy didn't mind doing the books. She liked numbers and was good at it. Mrs. Winston did all the rest and she did it exactly right.

In many ways, I was lucky. I took a part-time job in one of the clinics at the city hospital. That helped financially. In addition, Medicare had just started and many of those clinic patients had Medicare and later Medicaid. The clinic doctors made whatever Medicare or Medicaid paid, and that was additional income to our salary. Peggy did the horrendous job of completing all those insurance forms and getting payment. I would then evenly distribute that money to the staff.

Another source of income was the University Of Tennessee College Of Medicine resident staff that would send Medicare and Medicaid patients to me for hospital admission if those doctors found no medical problem of interest to them. Consequently, I would carry a hospital census of at least 30 patients at all times and several times my hospital census exceeded 40 patients. All those hospital patients required a lot of daytime and nighttime attention, but to a relatively young man beginning a practice it was relatively easy. This arrangement continued for six or seven years. I have forgotten why it slowed, however by that time I had a busy practice, so it didn't bother me.

I had another major advantage. I was the only board-certified endocrinologist in the surrounding hundreds of miles. The phenomenon of supply and demand was in place. Much of public had heard of endocrinology and metabolism, knew that it dealt with hormones and metabolism, and thought they might have a hormonal or metabolic cause for their problems. Consequently, they wanted to consult an endocrinologist; and they came to see me.

Another advantage was that I put my name in the Yellow Pages telephone book under PHYSICIANS as did all the other doctors. However, I also put my name under the new heading ENDOCRINOLOGY & METABOLISM. I was the only doctor listed there, because I was the only board-certified doctor in Endocrinology & Metabolism. That also increased my patient load considerably. The local medical society tried to stop me from listing under ENDOCRINOLOGY & METABOLISM, but I told them, at Peggy's suggestion, that it was against the law to restrict trade, and that I would contact the Federal Trade Commission if the medical society caused any more trouble. That was the last I heard about the listing. However, I know it made many local doctors furious, especially the generalists, who did not want subspecialists to come into the area and compete with their practice.

My practice monopoly continued for many, many, years. However, more and more endocrinologists moved into the area (just like fishermen who gather around the guy catching all the fish). I would have formed an endocrinology group, but the newer doctors were younger and, in my opinion, were not as well trained. There would have been some friction. In addition, third-party payers started paying much less to the front-line, cognitive (non-procedure) types of doctors such as Endocrinologists who make the diagnosis, but paid much more to the doctors who do a procedure.

Therefore, I thought it best to close my office and join a multispecialty group. The hours and the on-call arrangements were much better than my solo practice, and the income was quite adequate, because Peggy and I had done financially well over the years. In addition, I had more time to work on my diagnosis program.

Chapter 16 Still Trying to Change How Doctors Diagnose a Problem.

My new group used electronic medical records (EMR). When a patient had more than a routine problem, I would use my computerized diagnosis program, and paste the list of the more likely diagnoses on to the patient's EMR record where everyone could see it. My list would include instructions on how users viewing the list could find the program on their computer and copy the program for their own use. However, bottom line—almost nobody used my program or inquired about it.

The program certainly worked for me, and intuitively I assumed it would help other doctors (and their patients!). I can work up a patient more accurately and in one-tenth the time it takes other doctors. I can go directly to the problem just like Willy Sutton, the bank robber. (You know the story. When Willie was asked why he robbed banks, he replied, "Because that's where the money is.") Duh! The lists advise me on where the diagnosis is. Patient has a fever and chest pain? That's easy. Here is the list of my top 40 causes for fever and chest pain (I show these lists merely to imply that many doctors fall far short of considering the diagnostic possibilities, and to illustrate all the work and time I put into this program).

PROBLEM LIST:
FEVER, CHEST PAIN

40 more likely diagnoses for a large sample of patients having the above problem(s), the diagnoses being listed in their approximate order of probability.

RANK	DIAGNOSIS	SCORE
1	FEVER	100
2	INFECTION	95

```
3    VIRAL INFECTION              68
4    COMMON COLD                  65
5    INFLUENZA                    63
6    THYROIDITIS                  37
7    BACTERIAL INFECTION          35
8    LYMPHOMA                     35
9    BILIARY DISEASE              35
10   THYROTOXICOSIS               35
11   PNEUMONIA                    34
12   CONGEST.HEART FAILUR         32
13   APPENDICITIS                 32
14   PERICARDITIS                 31
15   ABSCES/LIVER/SUBPHRE         31
16   PULMONARY EMBOLISM           31
17   MALIGNANCY                   31
18   PERITONITIS                  30
19   TRAUMA                       30
20   HEMOLYSIS/HGBINEMIA          30
21   LUPUS ERYTHEMATOSIS          30
22   ANEURYSM                     30
23   CHEST TRAUMA                 30
24   HYPERVENTILATION SYN         30
25   NOXIOUS FUMES                29
26   PANCREATITIS                 29
27   ATRIAL MYXOMA OR TUM         29
28   SYPHILIS                     28
29   FAMILIAL MEDIT.FEVER         28
30   PERIARTERITIS NODOSA         27
31   MIGRAINE                     27
32   MYOSITIS                     25
33   HEART DISEASE                25
34   COSTAL CHONDRITIS            20
35   MED/DRUG REACTION            20
36   ESOPHAGITIS                  20
37   G.U.  INFECTION              16
38   GI/ABD IMAGING DEFEC         15
39   INFEC.MONO/E B VIRUS         15
40   PULMONARY DISEASE            15
     265 Diagnoses considered/ 40 Requested/ 40 Listed.
```

When examining a patient I can go down that list in a minute or two, ask the pertinent questions, do the pertinent exam, and order the pertinent tests and/or treatment. Done. Complete. Accurate. Within minutes. It is so simple and so easy that I'm afraid it angers some of my colleagues. Other doctors in our group need an hour to do such an extensive workup. However, time is money. Therefore, doctors are in a hurry and are forced to do a mediocre evaluation in five minutes. Those doctors have to throw a bunch of lab tests, EKGs, and imaging studies against the wall and hope something sticks that leads them to the correct diagnosis.

Well, in any case, my program readily solves the problem. However, no one seems to see its advantages. Its worth. The money and lives it would save. The doctor-caused diseases it would prevent. Oh, the simplicity of it. Patient has a problem? Look at the list. Establish the diagnosis. Then decide the treatment. One! Two! Three!

I gradually became leery of putting my list of differential diagnosis into the patient's electronic medical record. My colleagues and peers seemed to scoff at my lists, demean the program, and demean me for using it. In that situation, I am outnumbered by the ignorant. *When around fools, it is foolish to be wise.* Therefore, I frequently would click on my program, use my lists, but would not copy the lists to the patient's chart.

Chapter 17 Advantages of My Program Over Other Programs.

Sales for my diagnosis program finally stopped. I had not sold a program in a long time. The drop in sales would not have been so frustrating if similar programs were any better.

Many of those other programs were introduced with much fanfare, advertisement, and expense, *but they were not better.* In fact, they were and still are inferior to my program. Those programs are too complicated, have too many bells and whistles, or consume too much of the doctor's time. They have significantly fewer diagnoses, and the diagnoses are not listed in any order of probability but merely clumped together so a rare diagnosis (remember a zebra) is sometimes at the top of the list or right next to a common diagnosis (a horse). In addition, many programs take too long to run. They ask too many questions. If the user doesn't know the answer to the question (usually an unnecessary question), the entire program might be erased, and the user have to start over again.

Furthermore, those programs are too specific. For example, my program has ABDOMNAL PAIN. That's it! However, other programs have causes for UPPER ABDOMINAL PAIN or RIGHT UPPER QUADRANT ABDOMINAL PAIN or LEFT UPPER QUADRANT ABDOMINAL PAIN or LOWER ABDOMINAL PAIN or RIGHT LOWER QUADRANT ABDOMINAL PAIN or LEFT LOWER QUADRANT ABDOMINAL PAIN. The problem with that format is the doctor or the patient frequently cannot be that specific as to exactly where the pain is. Therefore, in my program I simply list "ABDOMINAL PAIN" no matter where the pain is in the abdomen. So quick, so simple, and more accurate, because some disorders of the abdomen can cause symptoms in the upper abdomen in some patients or in the lower abdomen in other patients. *Being too specific can cause the doctor to miss the diagnosis.* Again, my approach is to generalize, to surround the problem (in this example, abdominal pain), and then pursue the more likely causes at the top of the list. Keep it simple.

The same applies to arm pain. Some programs list UPPER

ARM, or LOWER ARM, or WRIST, or FRONT OF ARM, or BACK OF ARM, etc. Again, many times patients cannot tell exactly where the pain is located. Again, it is unwise to be too specific. Those other programs list all of those locations, whereas my program simply has, "UPPER EXTREMITY PAIN" and gives the list of causes arranged in a decreasing order of the most likely diagnosis. My program is easier, faster, inclusive, and more accurate.

As I mentioned, the lists of diagnoses in other programs are too short, and consequently they do not include many important diagnoses. For example, my program lists 188 causes for diarrhea. Other programs might list only 10 to 20 diagnoses. A critic might say my lists are too long. They are not too long. That is our job; to find the diagnosis, no matter how long the list.

Another advantage of my program is that many patients have more than one disorder e.g. obesity, fluid retention, hypertension, arthritis, etc. My program will consider those additional diagnoses. An example is a patient with low blood pressure and an elevated blood test suggesting an acute myocardial infarction (heart attack). However, that patient might have additional problems such as a severe infection or, as mentioned earlier, a rupturing aortic aneurysm. My program alerts the doctor to those additional diagnoses that might require immediate diagnosis and treatment.

To sum it up, my diagnosis program is far superior to those other diagnosis programs. So, it doesn't surprise me those other programs have limited sales, but it *does* surprise me that doctors don't use my program.

Chapter 18 Doctors Continue Their "Hit or Miss" Diagnosis.

Doctors consider the few diagnoses they can recall from memory and then order tests or give treatment. They hope the tests or treatment will prove their diagnosis. In essence, they are like car manufacturers who make the car buyer *test drive* the car. The car buyer is actually the quality control for the company. Similarly, if a patient gets better (car runs okay), the doctor (car manufacturer) is okay. If the patient continues to have a problem (car won't run), the patient goes back to the doctor (car dealer), in which case more tests and treatments (car shop) are tried (more expense and problems). If the doctors used my diagnosis program, they would be more likely to find the diagnosis the first time, not after numerous, possibly fatal *tune-ups*.

Don't get me wrong. Doctors are under a lot of pressure. They need to see many patients and to see them quickly. Consequently, they order a slew of tests, usually including a CAT scan or some other expensive study such as an MRI—or both—and hope the tests will uncover the correct diagnosis. However, the patient walks out of the office with the diagnosis (might or might not be correct), with the tests (might or might not be appropriate), and with the treatment (might or might not be the right treatment). In addition, the patient is generally happy with the encounter at least for the time being (about 30 percent of patients feel better purely from the placebo effect of the medications, the doctor visit, or the tests).

Why don't doctors use lists such as mine? One reason is that the doctor, tries to be a *take-charge* doctor. *Take-charge* doctors are impressive to patients, appear powerful, all knowing, and in control. They don't need any reference material. They say, "Oh yes," grimace as the patient describes the headache, and then look at the head and presses here and there. This takes only minutes. To the patient, the doctors' take-charge demeanor shows a sign of knowledge, strength, and control. The few minutes they spend with the patient merely joking or appearing deep in thought, looking enormously knowledgeable and in charge—all of that takes very little time.

Again, however, too often the tests are negative or wrong and too often the problems persist. This as a bad situation. The doctor then suggests the patient is under stress, blah, blah, and they order more tests, a different pain medication, and a tranquilizer. The patient is now on a slippery slope. The medications have significant side effects, many of which could make the patient feel even worse. If the patient is not better, then more doctoring, more pills, even surgery, or referral to a specialist who does the same thing and orders additional tests. Finally, somebody might come up with the correct diagnosis and do the right thing. However, the patient frequently has so many medication or surgical side effects by that time that the underlying initial cause of the problem is missed. So, more problems, more illness, more tests, and more treatments.

To review this fiasco (I know this is repetitious, but the point needs to be drilled in) the patient comes into the office. Dr. X greets the patient. The patient explains the symptoms; Dr. X will listen a bit and make a cursory exam, again being under considerable pressure to see the patient quickly (I'm always entertained when I see doctors listen to the heart and lungs through clothing, an impossible way to hear important abnormalities; or take blood pressure readings with the blood pressure cuff over a sleeve). Then the doctor will authoritatively ask a few questions, order some money-producing and malpractice-protecting tests (doctor needs income and protection), write out a prescription, and the doctor and the patient at least at that encounter are usually happy. However, if the patient is not one of the lucky patients who gets better, and the studies do not discover the correct diagnosis, the doctor, depending on the patient's tolerance and the severity of the problem, might proceed with some more history taking, physical examination, and additional tests and medications. Alternatively, the doctor might refer the patient to a specialist, who will do pretty much the same thing, except possibly, the specialist will have more knowledge and will arrive at the correct diagnosis. However, the specialists often take too much time to find the correct diagnosis, if they ever do, and even though their memory's list of causes might be more extensive than that of the referring doctor, the specialist's memory is still too often inadequate.

My point is that the doctor does not have an organized check-off list to help establish the most likely causes for the patient's problem. Without a proper list, the workup is helter-skelter, unfocused, and dangerous.

What can the patient or the doctor do to avoid that unhappy scenario? *Use my computer diagnosis program* or any similar program if there is one (I never could find one). Look at the first 40 diagnoses on the list. These are the more likely diagnoses. Just like Willie Sutton. Therefore, the doctor, when looking for the diagnosis, should look where the diagnosis is. In other words, look for the most common causes of the problem. All of this takes only a few minutes. When doctors know what they are looking for, they are much more likely to spot it. In addition, if the diagnosis is still illusive, then the doctor should review the original list and consider the next ten-or-so additional diagnoses down the list. The odds again are in favor of the diagnosis being there. If not, then the next ten should be considered. The doctor is homing in on the diagnosis, no matter how rare that diagnosis might be.

Again, in all fairness to doctors, powerful forces exist that cause them to act as they do. Certainly, their main goal is to help the patient and that alone can be daunting, frustrating, and difficult. However, other different and harmful obstacles interfere with the doctor's noble efforts. For example, the overhead expenses, not just for the usual office help, but also for the additional personnel to comply with the incessant and increasing regulations, to complete the codes, and to handle the insurance papers that inundate the office. Other expenses are the office personnel health insurance, the office personnel retirement plans, the rent, the malpractice insurance, dealing with mountains of paper work, arguing with HMOs, Medicare, Medicaid, Obamacare, PPO administrators and other third parties, lost claims, denied claims, unpaid claims, partial payment of claims, resubmission of claims, denial of necessary tests and procedures including surgeries, angry patients, litigious patients, threatening patients, and—sick patients. All of that can destroy any attempt by the doctor to help people. Many doctors become inured to the patient's problems. Some doctors cannot take the stress. This situation is not a happy one—for doctors or for patients. Again, make it easy on yourself, doctor. Use my diagnosis program!

Chapter 19 There Are Essentially Three Types of Medical Practice.

The practice of medicine used to be between the patient and the doctor. The doctor would see the patient, the doctor would order tests or start treatment, a follow-up would be arranged, and the doctor would bill the patient *for services rendered.* That was it. No third parties.

Now days you have the second type of practice where third parties such as hospitals, insurance companies, large corporations, etc., virtually control the doctors, control the patients, control the number of admissions, control the doctors' income, control the lab tests doctors can order, control the payment for the tests, control the surgery the doctors can do, control the payment for the surgery, control referrals to other doctors, control the number of patients the doctors are required to see, on and on. In addition, many third parties make the doctor pay for a large part of the expenses!

The doctors' income in this type of practice is usually as low as the doctors will tolerate. Moreover, those doctors must have happy and healthy patients—or, if they are employed by others—they can be fired. Bottom line: see large numbers of patients, keep them happy, healthy, and do it all at a minimum cost. This is not a pretty picture for the patient or the doctor. The doctor is obviously hurried and is consequently apt to make errors. In addition, patients who have more than a simple problem will tend to get less than the necessary attention and care.

The third type of practice is a newer type of practice called "concierge" practice. The patient pays up front for a specified type of coverage. The doctor does not honor any third party and deals only with the patient. That doctor can essentially do whatever the contract and the patient allow. Payment is arranged strictly between the patient and the doctor. If doctors know that money is no obstacle, they can spend more time with the patient, charge more, order more tests, and make a good profit. If the patient has paid little money up front, the doctor can easily, especially with my diagnosis program, adjust the workup and charges downward. The concierge doctor has the potential to make a large income, the limit being the amount of money paid up front and the number of such patients accepting the arrangement. In addition, the doctor need not contend with third party hassles.

As an aside, doctors who do surgery or expensive procedures can make much more money than the non-procedure doctors. For example, a doctor doing a 30-minute procedure such as a colonoscopy can be paid $1,000 whereas a doctor spending 30 minutes doing a history, a physical examination, and arranging for tests can possibly get about $200. In addition, this latter doctor needs to later discuss the test results with the patient and, if indicated, start a treatment. This takes at least another 15 to 30 minutes. So, the procedure doctor makes about $2000 per hour compared to $300 per hour for the non-procedure doctor. (Don't forget, a lot of this income goes to overhead.) Obviously, the procedure pays much better than ferreting out the correct diagnosis and starting the best treatment. The only way the non-procedure doctors can make a reasonable income is to require a higher fee for their time, and/or see lots of patients, which means seeing them quickly. The consequences are obvious.

I cannot help but emphasize that any of those doctors would benefit by using my diagnosis program. They can quickly analyze a patient and order what tests, surgeries, or whatever else best fits their practice, and give better care.

By the way, I do have to laugh at times at my colleagues. Once a month our medical staff would discuss a case of interest. One patient we discussed was obviously confused, didn't know where he was, refused intravenous fluids, medications, and tests, and kept saying he would not cooperate unless he were at so-and-so hospital. He was obviously so confused that I suggested to his doctor, whom I will call Dr. X, that he tell the patient he was indeed at that hospital, and maybe he would cooperate enough to start the necessary treatment. Dr. X quickly replied to our group, in a serious and admonishing voice, "I do not lie to my patients." So much for the art of medicine. At the next meeting, one of our staff related a problem for which that same Dr. X suggested that the other doctor *mislead the patient*. The staff doctor, in front of the staff, in a serious, admonishing, and loud voice said, "Dr. X--I do not lie to my patients." I threw a quick look at Dr. X. He looked the other way.

Sales for my computer program were nil. I could not believe it. Or accept it. My program offered great improvements to the delivery of health care. Yet—no takers. Doctors ignore it; and they continue to misdiagnose. What are those doctors thinking? Anyway, more down in-the-dumps times for me. However, I did not think of myself as a failure. On the contrary, I thought those other doctors were the failures (the typical defense mechanism). Nevertheless, facts are facts. No buyers.

Something nice caught my attention yesterday. It had rained a beautiful springtime shower. It was early in the morning. Some ferns on the patio had been blown over so I righted them.

As I stood up, a budding dogwood bloom brushed my cheek. It kind of said, "I am with you. No fear. I am with you."

Chapter 20 My Web Site.

I started a Web site. This was a new and exciting thought in that the Web site could benefit doctors and patients around the world. It would be a logical extension of my book and computer-assisted diagnosis program. Moreover, it would justify all of my work, hopes, and dreams.

The user would simply click on any symptom, sign, or test listed in the index, and would get a list of causes arranged in my usual decreasing order of probability. My Web site was the same as my computer program except only one symptom could be evaluated at a time, for example only WEAKNESS. (My computer program on the other hand could evaluate up to six symptoms at a time, example WEAKNESS, ABDOMINAL PAIN, HEADACHE, etc.

Producing this Web site took many additional hours of work. I had to get all of those headings and lists of diagnoses transferred to the Web site, and then to program it so a user needed only to click on a symptom.

I thought there would be millions of people who would want a prioritized list of causes for their symptoms, readily available, free, on the Internet. I included a link to the famed *Merck Manual* and to the National Institutes of Health Web site *PubMed*, both of which give in-depth information to doctors and lay persons about any of the disorders listed on my Web site.

After about three months, my Web site was launched. Sad to say, few people used it. I probably have used my computer program and/or the Web site hundreds of times over the past several years. Maybe a handful of others have used it during that time. Furthermore, no one has ever commented about my program or the Web site other than the few instances I have already mentioned.

Anyway, I continued to think my approach of using the program or the Web site was essential to being a good doctor. I said to myself, too bad other doctors did not like it. Therefore, I would try to improve it here and there, but in fact, the program needed no improvement. It was already complete and straightforward.

Again (I know, ad nauseam), a person has for example leg pain. Look at the list of causes for LOWER EXTREMITY PAIN, all causes neatly arranged in descending order of probability. Consider the more likely diagnoses at the top of the list. If no diagnosis is apparent, re-assess those diagnoses and look further down the list. Back and forth until the correct diagnosis is established. So simple, so effective, so easy, and so necessary. All of these advantages—and nobody does it. Over 800,000 doctors in the U.S.A., and only a relative small number bought my book or computer program, or used the free lists on my Web site.

Well, so far today some more hits (clicking on a web site is a *hit*). Early in the morning. I wonder if these hits are Asian and Middle Eastern users. It is wonderful, my program being used around the world! I know. I'm dreaming, but it is so much fun. Fantastic how the finding of more hits is exciting. I remember how it would send me through the clouds when I sold a book or a computer program. I would walk briskly and enthusiastically down the hospital halls, hailing my colleagues, happy and confident. Satisfied. Much better effect than any drug could possibly be, although I have nothing with which to compare it except the time when a dentist gave me a shot of something before doing some dental work. I did feel good after that shot, maybe only because the pain was gone. However, that good feeling was nothing compared to selling a book, a computer program or getting more hits.

The hits mean to me somebody has a problem, is in trouble, worried, or curious, trying to find the answer, and my Web site will help them: A tangible, initial, first step for them to establish the diagnosis. The Web site will give them the comfort of knowing an extensive search has been done. Personally, in my practice, I always know an extensive search has been done. I sleep well at night.

There is no argument that modern medical care can be proud of many things. For example, the CAT and MRI scans are incredible. They allow us to look into the body much better and safer than with a scalpel. Moreover, some of the medicines we use can result in miraculous cures. However, those machines and medicines only help to a limited extent. For example, ordering a CAT of the head for someone who has chronic headaches will miss more than half of the top 40 causes. Consequently, it is terrible that a doctor would rely almost solely on a CAT of the head, because, if the CAT is negative, the result too often is that doctors will diagnose only the more common causes that they can easily recall from memory, and treat the patient for one or more of those diagnoses. Doctors should use my lists; then they would be more able to make the correct diagnosis.

Chapter 21 Promotional Attempts. How to Cut the Health Care Expense by Billions of Dollars, Deliver Excellent Care, and Still Cover Everybody.

I got several more hits recently. Those hits were probably caused by two letters to the editor I sent to a well-known, nationally distributed newspaper. I described the advantages of computer-assisted diagnosis programs and how those programs could cut the cost of medical care in half. The hits were possibly the newspaper investigating my Web site. Here is one of those emails:

Dear Editor:

I agree with the February 23 Opinion Page commentary "Good Drug, Bad Customers - II," that it is difficult to understand why artificial intelligence software hasn't already relieved doctors of their responsibility for making a correct diagnosis.
Others and I sell these computer-assisted diagnosis programs, but few doctors use them, and worse, they scoff at them.

If doctors were limited only to testing for diagnoses that had a reasonable chance of being correct, the cost of medical care would be greatly reduced, the doctors' time would be better used, fewer unnecessary tests would be performed, and there would be fewer complications from those unnecessary tests/treatments. In addition, fewer incorrect diagnoses would be made, fewer correct diagnoses would be missed, fewer doctor-caused diseases would occur, and more treatments would be directed at the real diagnosis.

Sincerely,
David E. Wade, M.D.

However, the medical laboratories, medical device makers, pharmaceutical companies, doctors, and most hospitals (the medical-industrial complex) would undoubtedly make less money if doctors used such diagnosis programs. Maybe that is why the newspaper did not print my letter. The medical-industrial complex buys a lot of advertisement space.

I sent the second email to the editor of the same newspaper in response to another Opinion/Editorial page article. I emphasized that a major problem in medical care delivery is the need for some limitation as to what doctors are allowed to do. I emphasized that the cost of making the correct diagnosis would plummet—if the doctor were limited to looking for the *reasonable diagnoses*. I estimated the cost would be cut in half. Billions and billions of dollars would be saved. For example, rarely is there a reason for a doctor to get a CAT of the abdomen on the first or second visit, because it is seldom needed to diagnose the more likely causes of an abdominal problem. Has the doctor eliminated these possibilities before ordering the CAT? I doubt it. So, approximately $1,000.00 is saved right there. Multiply that by the millions of CATs of the abdomen, and that comes to billions of dollars. Furthermore, by using my program or Web site the correct diagnosis is more apt to be made, and made quickly, which is another saving of money and lives. Moreover, there would not be that additional expense of medical or surgical treatment for the wrong disease.

Here is that letter:

Dear Mr. XXXX:

I enjoyed reading your article in the BBBB.

In an attempt to improve health care and at the same time lower health costs, I humbly ask you to consider two ideas for future articles. The first concerns the premium, copay, and deductible that stop many patients from seeking medical advice even when they might benefit from it. After the deductible is met, many patients then "want the works", demanding many additional tests and treatments even though they might be inappropriate.

A solution might be to make the premium, copay, and deductible acceptably small, but to make any additional costs high enough to control over use. Then people will not hesitate to buy insurance or get the initial doctor opinion, but will aggressively question the need for additional doctor visits, tests, treatments, or surgery.

The problem is that some health providers unfortunately, wittingly or not, can easily convince patients that additional unnecessary or inappropriate tests, treatments, and surgeries *are indicated.*

The word *indicated* is the crucial word and leads to my second idea, the role of Computer-Assisted Diagnosis (CAD). CAD can limit the doctor to a list of diagnoses the doctor is authorized to pursue. Please click on http://computeassistdiagnosis.blogspot.com for an example of what CAD can do. Several CADs are available.

Doctors are less likely to order excessive tests/treatments/surgeries if they are limited to evaluating the more likely diagnoses, a list of say the top 40 diagnoses, and know they might be called to justify their decisions to order more.

Some of the cost savings made possible by enforcing computer-assisted diagnosis programs are:
1. The number of diagnoses to be considered can be adjusted up or down, thereby controlling costs.
2. The doctor can be held accountable for unnecessary tests/treatments/ surgeries.
3. Fewer tests lead to fewer false positive results. (False positive tests lead to missing the correct diagnosis, more testing, additional incorrect diagnoses, incorrect treatment, more illness, and more expense.)
4. Proceeding quickly to the correct diagnosis.
5. Almost 99.9 percent of diagnoses are made by the exclusion of the other possible diagnoses (few tests have 100 percent specificity and accuracy for a given diagnosis). Therefore, usually the only way to establish the correct diagnosis is to rule out the other possibilities. Such a list of diagnoses is large, but CAD will narrow down those diagnoses to the ones that are more likely correct.
6. Since medications frequently cause side effects, medications are frequently high

on the list. The result is fewer meds will be prescribed, which in itself would save billions of dollars.

I hope you consider this information useful.

Sincerely,

David E. Wade, M.D.

I received no response other than the editor's reply that Abraham Lincoln would have said it better. (In that regard, I recall an article by a noted authority who described dozens of grammatical and syntactical errors in the Gettysburg Address.) Anyway, I did get a few hits on my web site, but that was it. However, again remember—the medical-industrial complex pays a lot for newspaper ads.

I have tried countless ways to promote my programs. I have stacks and stacks of such information. Reams and reams of it. One productive method to promote my book and computer-assisted diagnosis program was a quarterly newspaper called *Carnrick Classified*, published by Carnrick Pharmaceuticals, Inc. This publication was free of charge to doctors in the U.S.A. and its U.S. Territories.

Carnrick Classified gave free space for doctors to list advertisements to sell, rent, and swap homes, bikes, cars— almost anything, including computers and computer programs. So, I listed my program there, four times a year, for years and years. Finally Carnrick Pharmaceuticals, Inc. was bought by another company and *Carnrick Classified* was no longer published. Nevertheless, it was good while it lasted. I sold lots of books and computer programs through *Carnrick Classifieds*.

I think you the reader have by now gotten my message. I am going to give just two more of my promotional attempts, mainly to emphasize the unrelenting attempts I made to get my book, computer-assisted diagnosis program, and my web site to be used by the medical profession and the public.

Here is one of the many promos I put on my Web site:

DIAGNOSIS
New version 17.0. Exclusively for Windows
"Satus est initius mederi quam fini." (It is better to doctor at the beginning than at the end.)   ERASMUS

Dear Doctor:

Simply click on a patient's symptom over the NET, on your PDA, or on your PC. Instantly you get diagnostic possibilities listed in scored, decreasing probabilities.

This program helps the doctor remember the causes for various symptoms, signs, and test results. Furthermore, it recalls the diagnoses in the approximate order of their occurrence. Therefore, the differences in the diagnostic possibilities are virtually as applicable to any medical or surgical practice, from the family physician or surgeon, to the ER doctor.

Such a diagnosis list has obvious advantages. For example, it reminds the user of the more likely diagnosis(es), adds direction and focus to a patient evaluation, intuitively suggests treatments that should be started soon, and helps the user to order only appropriate tests and treatments.

The algorithm is as follows: A patient reports having a symptom such as nausea. The diagnosis program will be asked to list in decreasing order of probability the causes for nausea. Here is the list (user has requested 40 possibilities):

PROBLEM LIST:
NAUSEA
40 more likely diagnoses for a large sample of patients having the above problem(s), the diagnoses being listed in an approximate order of probability.

RANK	DIAGNOSIS	SCORE
1	NAUSEA	100

2	WT. LOSS & ANOREXIA	95
3	ANOREXIA	95
4	GASTROENTERITIS	90
5	GASTRITIS	90
6	ESOPHAGITIS	90
7	HYPERCHLORHYDRIA	80
8	COMMON COLD	70
9	INFLUENZA	70
10	GI/ABD IMAGING DEFEC	50
11	CHRONIC ILLNESS	50
12	DIABETES MELLITUS	20
13	MED/DRUG REACTION	20
14	DIABETIC KETOSIS	20
15	INFECTION	15
16	BILIARY DISEASE	10
17	PEPTIC DISEASE	10
18	FOOD POISONING	10
19	PARALYTIC ILEUS	5
20	CONSTIPATION	5
21	APPENDICITIS	5
22	GASTROINTEST OBSTRUC	5
23	PSYCHIATRIC	5
24	GASTRIC DILATATION	4
25	FEVER	4
26	HIATAL HERNIA	4
27	MALIGNANCY	4
28	FRIGHT	3
29	HYPOTHAL-PITUIT.DIS.	3
30	EXCESSIVE SMOKING	3
31	MIGRAINE	3
32	HI INTRACRAN PRESSUR	3
33	UREMIA/NEPHRITIS	3
34	ANY ACUTE ILLNESS	3
35	DIZZY/VERTIGO	3
36	PYLORIC OBSTRUCTION	3
37	ALLERGY	3
38	PREGNANCY	3

```
39   DUMPING SYNDROME                        3
40   PANCREATITIS                            3
     172 Diagnoses considered/ 40 Requested/ 40
Listed.
```

In general, the program says that of 100 cases having nausea, the more likely causes will have the higher scores and the less likely causes will have the lower scores. Obviously, clinicians are more likely to be correct if they consider the higher-scored diagnoses. However, if the diagnosis remains elusive, the clinician: (1) reviews the higher-scored possibilities; and (2) considers additional, lower-scored possibilities.

Two of the major problems for practicing physicians is trying to remember the diagnostic possibilities and taking so long to do it. That is where DIAGNOSIS is of great help. To review: A patient reports nausea. The doctor considers the diagnoses listed for nausea, and accordingly asks a few pertinent questions, does a pertinent examination, orders the pertinent tests, and is finished with this initial workup all within minutes. If the diagnosis is still elusive, the doctor reconsiders the possibilities by looking over the list again. We doctors do this every day. Now we have a list to help us remember the possibilities.

Some skeptics have said, "But you give a list of possibilities; I want the one correct diagnosis." Those people are unrealistic. A computer cannot consistently pick one correct diagnosis. Other skeptics have said, "But you don't know the real incidence of the diagnostic possibilities, therefore your statistics are fallible." I agree. I don't know and nor does anyone else. The incidence will vary depending on the practice, the geographical location, the season, and a myriad of other differences. That is why the doctor should only use approximations. My statistics are approximations. They are based on many years of study, experience, and thousands of opinions and publications by innumerable experts in the medical/surgical field. Doctors merely need to know the approximate frequency of occurrence; then they can fine-tune the workup.

DIAGNOSIS is extensive. The program includes the diagnoses to consider for hundreds of the more important symptoms, signs, and test results (SSTs), for example weakness, vomiting, depression, chest pain, hyponatremia; totaling more than 1440 diagnoses. However, in contrast to other programs fewer correct diagnoses would be missed. DIAGNOSIS does not confound the user with laborious and time-consuming multiple questions, or arbitrary, ill-defined symptoms, physical findings, and disease processes. Furthermore, in addition to listing the diagnoses in a decreasing order of probability, DIAGNOSIS also gives a numerical score to each diagnosis. Consequently, the doctor can tell quickly and more accurately the likelihood of one diagnosis, for example a score of 90, compared to another diagnosis, for example a lower score of 20. DIAGNOSIS KEEPS IT SIMPLE.

Simply double click on Diagnosis, and then click on- or type in the Sx, S, or Test result. The user can make multiple entries to help narrow down the list of probable diagnoses. The list of diagnoses for the one entry (or more entries combined) will be produced within seconds. The list is easily printed to hard copy, copied to an electronic medical record, or sent to other destinations.

DIAGNOSIS was probably the first computer-assisted diagnosis program commercially available. DIAGNOSIS goes directly to the problem—the diagnosis. Also, available free on the Internet, are such sources as PubMed.gov or the Merck Manual (click here to see those sites) that describe the disease, diagnosis, treatment, and more. Keeping DIAGNOSIS minimized makes it available for instant, on the spot consultation. Many other programs such as Harrison's Textbook of Medicine and ICD/CPT codes are kept up to date and are inexpensively available on the NET or as PC programs. These too can be kept running minimized for immediate use.

DIAGNOSIS is available as follows:
1. 3.5-inch disk. Run from disk or drag-drop the DX folder to your hard drive. Multiple entries can be computed simultaneously. If you are not completely satisfied with DX, return the items within 30 days for a full refund. Price: $25.00
2. The Web. Receive a URL from which you can access the diagnostic possibility lists via the Internet. The user can simply click on the SST of interest. Only one entry can be computed at a time. The Merck Manual and PubMed.gov are linked for the user's convenience. Price: $20.00
3. PDA (for example Palm Pilot, Handspring, Pocket PCs). For those who have the facility to copy and tailor text files of lists to their palm top. The user can simply open the SST file of interest. Only one entry can be computed at a time. Price: $20.00 U.S. currency, check, or money order: payable to David E.Wade, M.D., and mail to the address below.

Updates (indicated as a new version) are made on the few occasions a significant, documented, new disease is described, or when significant program improvements are developed.

David E. Wade, M.D.
Author:
WADE'S DIFFERENTIALS: an aid to diagnosis, Astor-Honor Inc.,
    New York, 1971.
COMPUTER-ASSISTED DIAGNOSIS SYSTEM.
Board Certification, American Board of Medical Specialists:
    Internal Medicine. 1966
    Endocrinology & Metabolism. 1972

Here is another promo for my Web site (the reader need not read all of this—it is given here again only to demonstrate my attempts to help doctors and their patients).

DIAGNOSIS/DX: Computer-Assisted Diagnosis

New version 17.0. Exclusively for Windows

"Satus est initius mederi quam fini." (It is better to doctor at the beginning than at the end.)   ERASMUS

Dear

Doctor:
Simply click on a symptom over the internet, on your PDA, or on your PC. Instantly you get the diagnostic possibilities listed in scored, decreasing probabilities.

As you know, trying to remember the causes for a symptom, sign, or test result is time-consuming and often impossible. The computer-assisted diagnosis program DIAGNOSIS/DX can help you remember these diagnoses, will list them for you, and it will list them in their approximate order of decreasing probability as seen in a general medical practice.

Giving consideration to the diagnosis list takes only a minute or two; extremely fast considering the myriad of possible diagnoses for any given symptom.

ACTUAL CASE:

   An elderly female patient presented with a subacute onset of psychosis, diarrhea, erythematous rash, and hyponatremia.

Differential Diagnosis for following problems: ENCEPHALOPATHY, DIARRHEA, ERYTHEMA, HYPONATREMIA

30 more likely diagnoses for a large sample of patients having the above problem(s), the diagnoses being listed in an approximate order of probability.

RANK	DIAGNOSIS	SCORE
1	MED/DRUG REACTION	165

```
2    VIRAL INFECTION        135
3    HYPONATREMIA           126
4    DIARRHEA               126
5    ENCEPHALOPATHY         100
6    MENOPAUSAL SYNDROME     98
7    PSYCHIATRIC             95
8    INTESTINAL INFECTION    90
9    GASTROENTERITIS         90
10   THYROTOXICOSIS          90
11   ALCOHOL                 67
12   CARCINOID               66
13   BACTERIAL INFECTION     65
14   IRON DEFICIENCY         63
15   UREMIA/NEPHRITIS        61
16   DUMPING SYNDROME        61
17   LIVER DISEASE           61
18   HYPOGLYCEMIA            61
19   CONGEST.HEART FAILUR    60
20   PANCREATITIS            60
21   ADRENAL INSUFFICIENC    59
22   INAP.ADH SYNDROME       57
23   MALIGNANCY              57
24   MALNUTRITION            57
25   CUSHING'S               56
26   PHEOCHROMOCYTOMA        56
27   PELLAGRA(B 2/NIACIN)    55
28   LYMPHOMA                55
29   LUPUS ERYTHEMATOSIS     55
30   INSECT/SNAKE BITES      55
```
     564 Diagnoses considered/ 30 Requested/ 30
Listed.

DX: PELLAGRA.

The IADH syndrome was probably due to her encephalopathy.

All of the problems rapidly cleared after starting niacin and temporarily limiting her fluid intake (IV fluids were started by the admitting doctor). She turned out to be a delightful, energetic patient who had been living alone and who had neglected her diet.

DIAGNOSIS/DX is extensive .... *(The promo continues here and is essentially the same as the many other promos I put on my website.)*

I remember writing letters to DIGITAL, IBM, Data General, and many others. I practically pleaded with them to use my ideas. No responses. I laughingly tell my friends how IBM made two mistakes: (1) They gave DOS back to Bill Gates; and (2) IBM ignored my program. I emailed Bill Gates. Nothing. I have mailed or emailed many medical clinics and hospitals. Virtually nothing. I would email doctors (hundreds of them) about my Web site. The utility of my programs is as obvious as $2 + 2 = 4$, but no takers. Virtually none of them responded.

I even tried some chat-room type advertising, recommending my program to some people who inquire on the internet about their symptoms. I even contacted the New York Yankees, suggesting they look at my site regarding one of their star player's illness. No hits. (I was right about the diagnosis.)

I submitted an ad in the Journal of the American Medical Association and in the American Medical News.

I attended a dinner for nurse practitioners, and emailed their president about the advantages of my computer program. I even sent a disk to her. She responded enthusiastically, saying she liked the program, would tell her group about it, and asked if she could make copies for her nurses. I agreed. That is the last I heard from them. No sales. No inquires.

Insurance companies and Health Maintenance Organizations were contacted. One intuitively would think they would want to limit expenses. What a good way for them to save money. They could limit payments only for those tests and surgeries that had a reasonable chance of helping the patient. However, I have since learned insurance companies, HMOs and the like, get a bill, pay it (unless someone doggedly complains about it), then ask for, and get incredibly higher premiums. It still doesn't make sense. You would think they would eventually price themselves out of the business; that their clients would go elsewhere. Evidently, that does not happen and the cost of health care continues to soar.

I finally joined a large hospital group that gave me even better hours, more paid holidays, and sick leave. Again, the pay was quite adequate.

Chapter 22 Discouraged

After all of this and dreadfully little response, I finally gave in. Ups and downs. Life is a roller coaster. I was for a long time, years in fact, down about my diagnosis programs. I could not believe it was ignored. Terrible. Again, what were these doctors and patients thinking?

I almost have to laugh when I consider all of my efforts. I remember one doc telling me the only guy who benefits from publishing anything is the guy who wrote it. That seems to be the truth. Those programs have been of tremendous benefit to my patients and to me, but evidently to almost no one else.

However, looking back on my life, I realized how lucky I have been. I have never suffered any serious disease—never— aside from those years with that bum ankle. Yet I feel bad about the problems patients have. I cannot fully appreciate the fears, loneliness, worry, and depression diabetics have when their toe is easily injured and infected from an injury that would cause only a minor problem to a nondiabetic. Those patients have found over time that little of what they do results in the toe being cured, and even if it does get better, it won't be long until the toe is infected again. They limp. They try to do their job, to work and to play like the rest of us. Yet, it cannot be done. If they do run and play, the toe problem comes back or gets worse. They are told to eat and exercise properly, test their blood more often, not to exercise too much (*but do enough*), on and on. In addition, the pressure from their family and from their doctor to maintain perfect control, so-called tight control; it suffocates them. They hardly can live without some worry that they are not doing as much of what they should be doing. They feel guilty and then angry. Tough!

And how about the husband or wife who loses their dear loved one? Their buddy. Their standby. Their honest, dedicated, friend. Terrible. Cruel. Hard to believe it is allowed.

Or patients with heart disease. They feel okay now, but they and their loved ones know it all could be over in a minute. Waiting for the other shoe to drop. Or the patients who think their cancer is gone but also fear it might come back. A new ache causes concern. A real worry. A worry they cannot suppress.

Oh, the stress and the worry we endure. I wish I had a remedy. My only remedies are: 1) avoid traffic accidents and falls, 2) advise women to get mammograms, do self-examination of the breasts, and get PAP smears, 3) do the colonoscopies if definitely indicated, 4) don't smoke, 5) maintain normal weight, and 6)having a bad memory helps. Do those things and look on the bright side. Then the rest is *whatever will be, will be.*

I sometimes wonder if I am out of touch. Maybe seriously out of touch. I remember the story about Dr. Semmelweis, who in the mid-1800s, tried to convince the medical establishment that puerperal fever, a deadly infection occurring during or shortly after delivery, was due to a bacterial infection and could be prevented by using sterile techniques. That doctor knew of hundreds of mothers who died from that infection, but no one would heed his advice. No one would listen. He eventually suffered from severe depression. (I remember a case of puerperal fever I was asked to treat during my internship. Ohhhhh—she was sick! However, she pulled through.)

I could tell that Peggy had finally given up on any chance that my endeavors would gain popularity or recognition. I would comment sometimes to her about my program or Web site, but she would keep doing whatever she was doing and not make a response. She acted as though she didn't even hear me. I can't blame her. Even I tired from any hope of my programs being used.

I have struggled with this endeavor for over 40 years. Yet, the use of my program and Web site has been virtually zero. Today is a down day. No hits so far. Peggy had two dental caps get loose, caused by her previous tumor irradiation. The irradiation also caused the problem of Peggy not being able to open her mouth widely. Consequently, the dentist and Peggy will have a difficult time. As Queen Elizabeth would say, deas horribils—not a good day.

However, there will be better days. Days when I'm happy, indeed ecstatic. I'm lucky in that my exhilaration comes from many sources: seeing my diagnosis program do its job, doing exercises at the office, practicing my golf swing by hitting little whiffle balls in my back yard, oil painting, playing a few holes of golf on my way home from the office, scraping a side of our house in preparation for painting, painting it, looking at my completed paint job, and walking around the yard figuring out how to put various hoses together in a masterful array of connections so Peggy and I can water the flower beds, tomatoes, ferns, and fill buckets with water for this and that. Our alfresco on our patio, a drink, twinkling lights hung from some dogwood branches overhead. Neat.

Hitting my practice golf balls is perfect entertainment. If I'm a little at loose ends, I go out to my makeshift tee area and hit some whiffle balls. Not much exercise, but fun. To hit the ball solidly and straight is a challenge and something physical. Or music. I have recorded dozens of tapes of the Saturday afternoon Metropolitan Opera broadcasts. You want to feel good? Listen to Verdi's "Va Pensiero" from Nabucco, or Puccini's "Nessiun dorm" (I admit checking on the spelling) from Turandot. Oh, I forgot popcorn. So good. Walk around the yard with a bowl of that.

No hits so far today. So depressing. I admit that I repeatedly keep going over all of this (Dr. Simmelweis?), but I still cannot understand why the lay public, let alone the medical community, is not interested in using a diagnosis program, especially my program. Certainly, for example, if a patient continues to have depression or weakness, especially after having been seen by a doctor, you would think the patient would go to the Internet and consult a diagnosis program. However, that does not seem to happen; I have seldom heard of a patient consulting the Internet for the cause of a symptom. They seem to consult it for treatments, read up about a diagnosis such as a cancer or high blood pressure, but seldom to investigate a symptom. However, last night Peggy and I saw an actor on a TV show click onto "Dr.Diagnostic.com" to find the causes for disorientation and headache. Maybe that will encourage the lay public to use a diagnosis program. Such an endorsement.

It has been about two weeks after writing the above. Only a few hits on my Web site. Hard to take, but facts are facts.

I do want to relate here a wonderful story. This is a good break. Several days ago, the *Wall Street Journal* had an article about the Yankee Stadium's field announcer, Mr. Bob Shepaard, the legendary "Voice of the Yankees." He is the gentleman who introduces the lineups before the game and also announces the player's name each time the player comes to bat. Mr. Shepaard and Mr. Mickey Mantle were to be guests on a morning TV show, and the script was for Mr. Shepaard to introduce Mickey as if Mickey were coming to bat at Yankee Stadium. The announcer, in his sonorous voice, as he had done those many years at Yankee Stadium, was to say, "The batter— Mickey Mantle." Mickey was not aware of the script so when he walked into the room, he was surprised to see Mr. Shepaard, and joked, "What's going on here? Were they afraid I wouldn't show up?" Mr. Shepaard said, "No Mickey. I'm here only to introduce you as I did those many exciting years at Yankee Stadium when you would step into the batters box to bat." Mickey paused then said, "Oh—ya know—I always got the shivers when I heard you say that." Mr. Shepaard responded, rather sadly, "So did I, Mickey. So did I."

I well remember the last time I had shivers. It was when I attended a funeral of a young soldier killed in Iraq. Incredible. Killed. Finality. Doing his duty. He was proud of being in the Army. A smart, scholastic guy. He had left a full scholarship at The Citadel to join the Army. He was the son of one of my hospital acquaintances who had earlier told us her son was in Iraq. We were impressed, but none of us thought he would be *killed*! But he was. Killed in combat. The day of the funeral was sunny, breezy—pretty. Many flags and admirers. And his mother.

Maybe, some day, doctors will start to use a diagnosis aid such as mine that lists the most likely diagnoses in a decreasing order of probability. It seems to me they *must* use it. It seems to me there is no alternative, unless we some day, can alter our brain in such a way to recall these diagnostic possibilities purely from memory—a brain transplant maybe. Until then, I have (still have) high hopes that a diagnosis program will make it into the mainstream of a doctor's practice.

ABOUT THE AUTHOR

Dr. Wade graduated from the Mount Healthy Public School System, Denison University, and the University Of Cincinnati College Of Medicine. His General Rotating Internship was at the University of California Service San Francisco General Hospitals, his Residency in Internal Medicine at Ohio State University Hospitals, and his National Institutes of Health Fellowship in Endocrinology and Metabolism at Creighton University School of Medicine Hospitals. He authored *Wade's Differentials, an aid to diagnosis*, Astor Honor, New York, NY, and developed the computerized diagnosis program, *DX Reminders*. Dr. Wade has been in medical practice for more than a half century.